POSITION
SEX

QUIVER

CONTENTS

Maybe your bedroom fare means a limited menu of Missionary and "doggy" style. You know there's more out there to savor, but experimenting with new recipes is a daunting thought, especially when your staples satisfy. Or maybe your sexual repertoire contains variations on old favorites, but they still lack a certain spice. Either way, *Position Sex* cooks up creative ways for you to turn up the heat in your bedroom!

Of course, there's no one precise recipe for great sex, because too many variables come into play. But one thing is for sure, experimentation can awaken your libido and bring more excitement to your lovemaking. All it takes is some concerted energy on the part of both lovers, a healthy amount of trust, and open communication.

Sounds easier than it looks? Well, before embarking on a diet of the new and exciting positions presented here, first consider the following areas that can help pave the way to erotic enlightenment. Self-awareness, understanding, and knowledge about sexuality are elemental ingredients of exquisite sex. Most sex therapists agree that fantastic sex does not come naturally, but requires some work.

1. COMMUNICATE. Trusting your partner will lead to open lines of communication.

2. EXPLORE. Forget every negative thing you were ever told about masturbation.

3. PAMPER. Combine this with exploring one another and you've got a potent combination for deepening your relationship inside-and outside-of the bedroom!

4. EXPERIMENT. Now we're making the move to more adventurous lovemaking!

5. ADD PROPS. Bring erotic stories, vibrators, and light bondage paraphernalia into the bedroom and you'll introduce a whole new dimension of pleasure to your sex life.

6. EXERCISE. Exercising will enhance your time in the sack, and in more ways than you may imagine.

7. UP THE FREQUENCY. Finally, trial and error is your friend, and of course, balance is key.

It's well within your power to transform your sex life from simple to sublime. Now feast your eyes on the fifty mouthwatering options, and remember: vanilla is just one of many flavors to savor!

1 • LOCK & LOAD

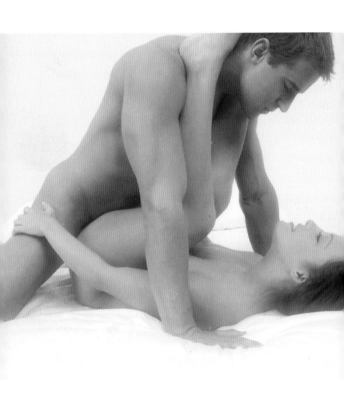

From the missionary position, she pulls her legs in toward her chest, extending them so that her ankles hook on his shoulders. He uses his hands to support both of their weight. Being extra flexible will allow both of you to enjoy the deep penetration and intense intimacy of this variation on your favorite standby. This position is great for a man with a shorter penis; however, if he is well endowed, thrusting can be painful for her, so be sure to communicate so you're both plunging to a pleasing depth.

WHAT'S IN IT FOR HER
When you draw your knees to your chest it shortens and tightens the vagina, so even shallow thrusts will make you tingle all over! Make sure to engage in ample foreplay, because your man won't be able to hold out for long! Try grabbing his hind-quarters to pull him deeper into you.

WHAT'S IN IT FOR HIM
This position is all about deep penetration and when your woman thinks you can't get any deeper, you lean forward and . . . WOW! Your balls will rest against her ass, pleasantly stimulating an often ignored area. Placing pillows beneath her bottom can also heighten your pleasure.

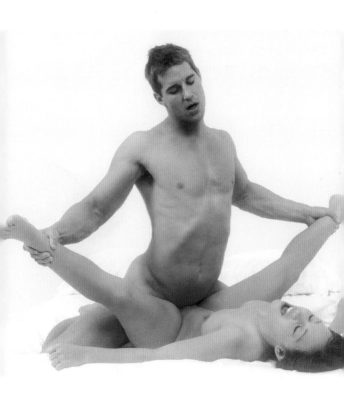

The woman lies on her back. The man kneels and enters her, holding a firm grip on her ankles and spreading her legs as wide as they comfortably can go. You'll want to experiment with the most pleasing width and pace of thrusting, because sensations can vary quite a bit.

WHAT'S IN IT FOR HER
In this position, you will likely fulfill one of his longtime fantasies, so revel in the fact that you are the star of the show. Penetration is deep and the pressure of his pelvic bone on your clitoris will add delicious friction to the mix.

WHAT'S IN IT FOR HIM
The turn-on for you will be seeing yourself insert your erect penis into her wet and willing vagina. The capability of men to become highly aroused from visual stimulation is well documented. Your lover will find immense gratification in knowing you're appreciating her naked and wide open body.

3 • THIGHS WIDE SHUT

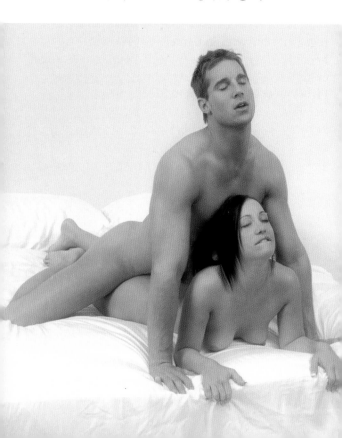

Lying face down on the bed, the woman rests on her elbows, with her legs parted just enough so that when her lover lies on top of her, he can slip inside. This can take some coordinated effort on both her and his part. Once he's in, she squeezes her legs together. (For an even tighter grip, she can cross her ankles!) He supports himself with his arms and either keeps them extended for more exaggerated thrusting or lowers down to his elbows for some front-to-back skin contact and rhythmic, rocking action.

WHAT'S IN IT FOR HER

This position is perfect for deep thrusting. It's relatively mellow in terms of motion, but you'll generate lots of friction with your legs closed tight. The squeezing will make the vagina feel longer and snugger and the combo of lying face down and contracting the thighs will stimulate the clitoris, which all but guarantees a stronger orgasm!

WHAT'S IN IT FOR HIM

The pure, animalistic lust of rear-entry sex combined with the extra tightness of your lover's vagina makes this one for the record books.

4 · BANANA SPLIT

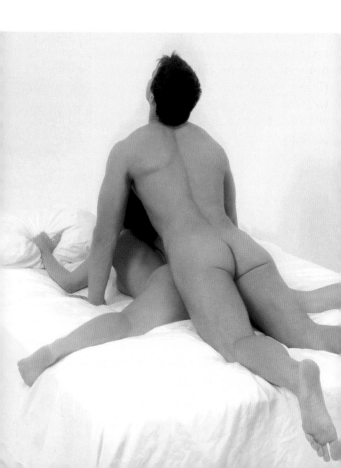

The woman lies face down on the bed, resting on her elbows. Once her lover slips inside, she slides her legs out very wide, so that they are almost perpendicular to her torso. He can remain higher up, supporting himself with extended arms, or drop down onto his elbows for extra contact. (If he lowers down, he needs to make sure the weight is comfortable for her. It's hard to get excited when you're being crushed!) For an added jolt, she can loosen and tighten his PC muscles to alternate sensations for him.

WHAT'S IN IT FOR HER

Extra-deep penetration and the feeling of friction on your pubic bone will send a spine-tingling jolt throughout your body, as both your G-spot and clitoris receive attention. Suggest a sexy mutual massage with oil before maneuvering into this position to add a sweet, slippery sensation.

WHAT'S IN IT FOR HIM

In this position, you will get to go deep, deep, deep while getting an amazing view of her backside. If she feels comfortable with you exploring her nether regions, you can get an added thrill out of teasing and fondling her anus.

5 • RUMP ROMP

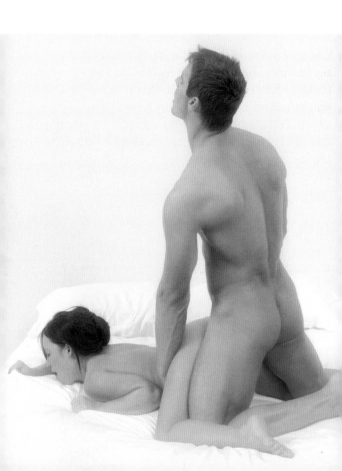

She lies on her stomach or on all fours, while her lover kneels behind her. He either places his legs inside or outside of hers and then enters her from behind. It can take some mutual experimentation to find the easiest entry into her vagina. If she wishes, she can close or tighten her legs to increase the friction and grip on his penis. He can thrust as slowly or as quickly as he likes and either grab her hips or reach around and play with her breasts and clitoris. The angle of penetration means the man can stimulate the upper inside wall of the vagina, where the G-spot is located!

WHAT'S IN IT FOR HER

This position allows for deep penetration. His penis will likely stroke your G-spot, which bodes well for you achieving vaginal orgasm. Your lover can also easily access your clitoris and play with it during sex for some added ecstasy.

WHAT'S IN IT FOR HIM

Rear entry sex takes a man back to his lustful roots. Seeing her ass, with her cheeks parted and your penis entering and withdrawing is almost too much stimulus for you! You will be uber-excited when taking her in from the rear, so don't be surprised if you come more quickly.

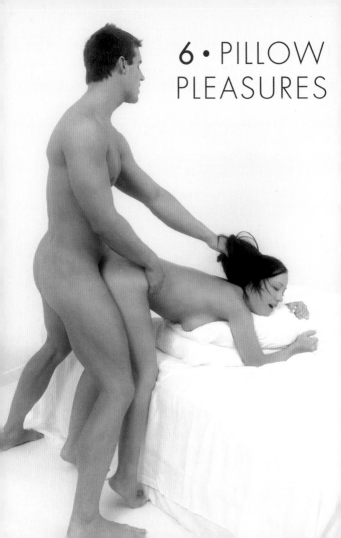

6 · PILLOW
PLEASURES

This hot, lusty position is akin to RUMP ROMP—on steroids! Take the action off the bed and onto the floor as he worships her sexy body. The setup is simple: Make sure one or two pillows are available. She stands on the ground and bends over the bed leaning onto the pillows. The man faces the woman's back, comes right up next to her with his legs slightly wider than hers, and enters her from behind.

WHAT'S IN IT FOR HER

This position will free up his hands to fondle your back and belly, massage your clitoris, gently tug your hair. . . . You'll want to incorporate lots of foreplay, because he may not be able to hold out for long. In addition to providing much-needed cushioning, the pillow can muffle your inevitable cries of ecstasy.

WHAT'S IN IT FOR HIM

With feet firmly planted on the floor, you will thrust with ease, control the tempo, and penetrate your lover oh-so-deeply! If you angle yourself up, your balls will rub against her hind quarters each time you make contact—an added jolt of pleasure!

7 · SIT'N'SPIN

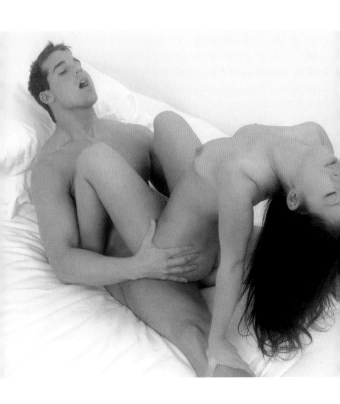

The man lies on his back, while the woman slowly squats onto his erect penis, positioning her feet near his hips and keeping her legs bent. (Be careful not to apply all of your weight at once!) She controls the action by moving up and down, gently rocking forward and back, or gyrating her hips in a circular motion. Up the erotic ante . . . by spinning around! She slowly rotates to the side and uses her hands and feet to keep herself stable. She then spins another 45 degrees so that her back is facing her man. She can either finish off in this position or continue to rotate around so that their erotic encounter comes full circle!

WHAT'S IN IT FOR HER

In this position, you will call all the shots and decide the tempo. Penetration is deep, but you can also experience feel-good friction as you rotate around. This 360-degree delight will stimulate all the different areas of your vagina!

WHAT'S IN IT FOR HIM

You will be able to sit back and enjoy the show or participate by using your hands to explore and caress, fondle and pinch, stroke and stoke her flame!

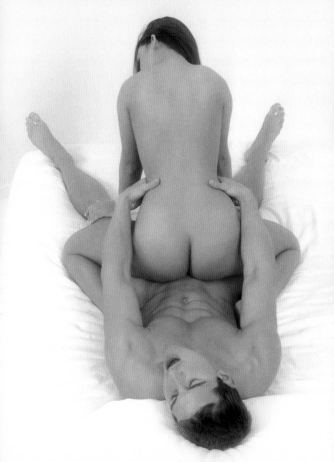

In this position, you will experience the tight fit of woman-on-top sex with the extra sizzle of doing it from behind! The man lies on the bed with outstretched legs. When he's ready, she squats over him with her back to him and slides onto his hard penis. With knees splayed around his torso, she places her hands on his legs and takes her man for the ride of his life!

WHAT'S IN IT FOR HER

This is one of the best ways for you to reach orgasm during sex, because you determine the rhythm, speed, and depth of thrusting during the session. His penis will penetrate the front of your vaginal wall, which means you're in for some yummy G-spot stimulation. You can also access your own juicy bits as well as his prized privates!

WHAT'S IN IT FOR HIM

Aside from the amazing view of her hot behind, your hands will be free to roam, caress, fondle, and feel your lover up in any way that you please!

9 · BODY SURFING

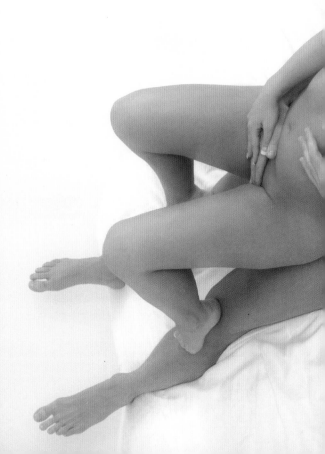

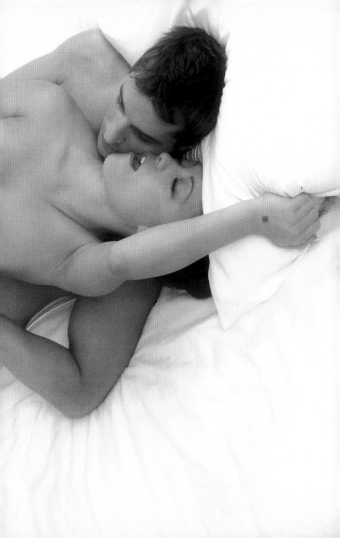

9 · BODY SURFING

The man lies on the bed with outstretched legs, while the woman faces his feet and slowly lowers herself onto his erection. This balancing act requires a lot of coordination! With his guidance, she lies back until she rests on her lover's chest with her cheek near his. He will get the awesome sensation of her vagina lengthening as she lowers down on him. Slowly and steadily, she pulls her feet up onto his legs, and you both ever-so-gently rock together to orgasm. This position is all about the deep feelings of small movements; he won't be able to move his pelvis, or she'll come apart.

WHAT'S IN IT FOR HER

You've got to be flexible to pull this position off, but when he penetrates you with your back to him, his penis will wake up different regions of your vagina. There's also plenty of skin contact, which will send chemicals in the pleasure center of your brain soaring.

WHAT'S IN IT FOR HIM

If you are both balanced, you will be free to focus your hands on her breasts and exploring her clitoris. When she orgasms, you'll feel the amazing throb of her anus, because your member will be close to the wall of her vagina—an unforgettable erotic experience!

10 · OCTOPUSSY

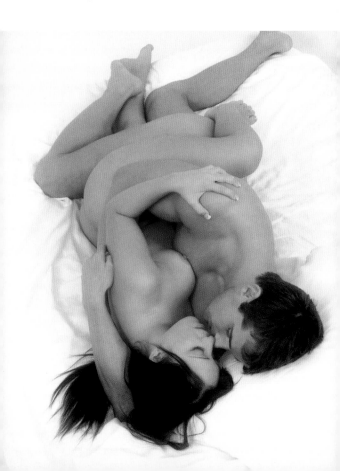

Here's a position perfectly suited for a long, slow, burning lovemaking session! The woman faces her man, and when heavy petting brings them both to the point of wanting to have intercourse, she moves in and opens her legs just enough for him to enter by slinging a leg over hers. Another option for getting into this position: They start in missionary and then they roll onto their sides, maintaining penetration as they rotate around. Enjoy the close and intimate feelings of making love while connecting with your eyes.

WHAT'S IN IT FOR HER

Here's a great way to delay orgasm: Tease your man by pulling your hips back almost to the point where his penis will come out and then plunge forward with a controlled thrust! The options for pleasure are only limited by your imagination . . . nothing is off-limits!

WHAT'S IN IT FOR HIM

If you're lucky, she'll send you over the edge by wandering to your perineum, the ultra-sensitive erogenous zone between your penis and anus. In this position, you can thrust gently and last for a long time before you come.

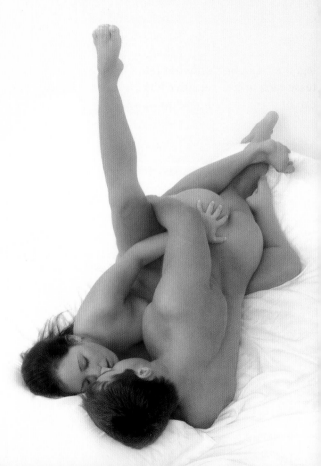

Time to show off your high kick! In this position, the man and the woman are on their sides facing one another. She lifts her top leg high into the air and guides his erect penis into her wet vagina. He slides inside and wraps his top knee around her leg. Both of your hands are free to fondle and tease each other's sensitive bits. See how long you can hold the position before your leg tires!

WHAT'S IN IT FOR HER

This side-by-side, intimate position is ideal for slow romantic lovemaking. The man can kiss and nibble your breasts, and you will see him do it—a powerful erotic stimulus!

WHAT'S IN IT FOR HIM

You can thrust gently and last for a long time before you come—movement of your hips is slightly restricted, but you can achieve good penetration. There is no danger of slipping out while you thrust, because your partner can wrap her leg around you and hold you inside of her while you make love.

12 • GIFT WRAP

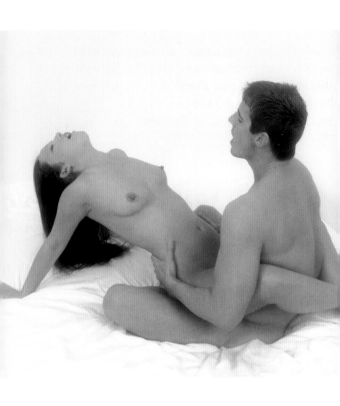

The man sits comfortably in a cross-legged or lotus position, and the woman lowers herself onto his lap, wrapping her legs firmly around his waist and hooking her ankles in the back. She then slides onto his erect penis and slowly leans backward onto her outstretched arms. Don't speed through that last part, because there's a chance she can hurt her man, he can slip out, or both. When successfully executed, you'll both feel a tight, albeit shallow, penetration.

WHAT'S IN IT FOR HER

Your man will rock you back and forth with a mesmerizing rhythm! You can vary the angle, reclining until you stop on a spine-tingling sensation. Your man can also hold you in place with one arm and use the other to roam the front of your body—including your clitoris!

WHAT'S IN IT FOR HIM

She will control the angle of penetration while you control the thrusting. Watch the temperature sky rocket as you pull her into you with great force just as you're about to come. This can fuel your animal instincts and heighten the intensity of orgasm for both of you!

13 · CROUCHING TIGER

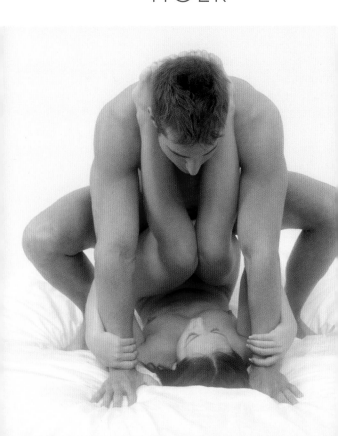

After an enthusiastic round of foreplay, she lies on her back, and while keeping her legs relatively tight, she pulls them up toward her chest and into her body. Imagine a jungle scene as the man suddenly—and gingerly—crouches over her, places his hands on the bed near her head, and slides into her. She hooks her ankles around his neck and grabs his arms for added leverage and support. For a wild ride, she can lift her ass to meet him for even deeper penetration. (For easier entry, she can put a pillow under her bottom.) You can rock, but keep in mind that movement is mostly deliberate and controlled in this intense lovelock.

WHAT'S IN IT FOR HER

If you're looking to connect in a carnal way, look no further. In this position, vigorous thrusting is abandoned in favor of slow, powerful contact. The angle of penetration means your man's bod will press against your vulva region—adding to your excitement!

WHAT'S IN IT FOR HIM

Because the woman is in a vulnerable position, you will have the ultimate control in this dominant position. As part of this scenario, you can tease her by partially withdrawing for a few shallow thrusts, followed by a deep and forceful stroke.

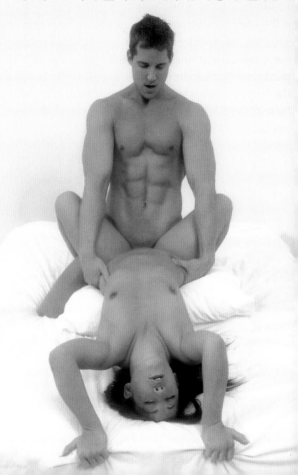

VIEW MASTER starts out in the basic missionary position, but for hotter results, the man places a pillow beneath the woman's ass to raise her up. This allows for deeper penetration. The woman places her head close to the edge of the bed. Once he's pumping, she lifts her arms and grasps the edge of the bed for added leverage. The motion of it will turn him on, and she'll get a slight head rush, making her extra tingly and amping up her excitement.

WHAT'S IN IT FOR HER

Pushing against his pelvis will add friction to the equation. When your man is supporting your ass during thrusting, he can apply a gentle pressure to draw your cheeks away from your anus and perineum, introducing a whole new erogenous zone!

WHAT'S IN IT FOR HIM

This will afford delicious, deep penetration, but only if you have a larger than average penis or a flexible erection. A man with a smaller penis will relish the sexy sight of shallow bobbing in her wet and willing vagina.

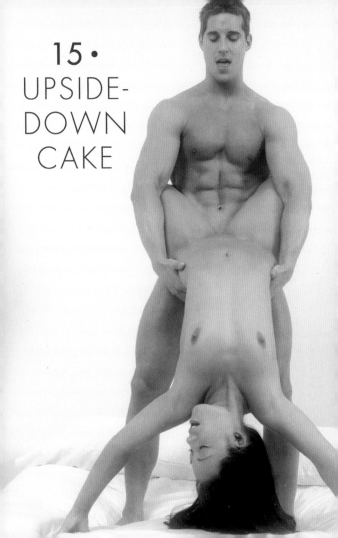

15 •
UPSIDE-
DOWN
CAKE

There are two ways to get into this amazing position: HARD—From VIEW MASTER, the man moves one leg so that it's bent and flat on the bed. Slowly, he pushes off that leg and rises up to a standing position, all the while keeping a firm grasp around her waist and maintaining penetration. Her hands are flat on the bed. When he's fully standing, she'll be in a backbend. HARDER—She lies on the bed with knees bent, arms overhead, and hands placed by her ears. She arches her back and brings her hips up high. The man kneels inside of her legs with one foot flat on the bed and grasps her around the waist to support her. When they're comfortable and ready, he raises up and lifts her off the ground, while he gently enters her.

WHAT'S IN IT FOR HER

This position means more than showing off your fitness—it represents an intimacy. In order to pull it off, you and your man must trust each other and be in tune with each other. The result will be a mind blowing orgasm for you, as the blood flows to your head and your G-spot is stimulated.

WHAT'S IN IT FOR HIM

This acrobatic position allows you to show off your prowess. But if she isn't ready, plant the seed in her head and then schedule a yoga class. Make it a point to practice together!

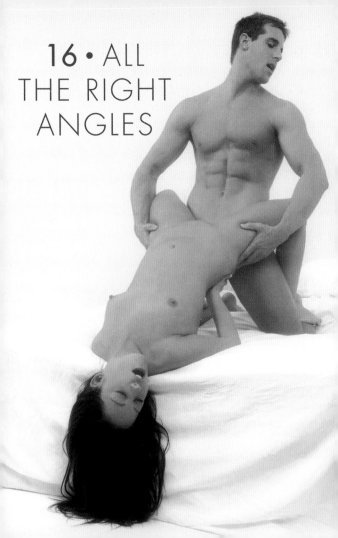

16 • ALL THE RIGHT ANGLES

She lies down on her back with her legs bent and apart and her arms bent behind her shoulders. When the man is ready to enter her, he positions himself between her knees and raises her hips to meet his pelvis. She pulls herself up using her hands to support her raised back. To up the erotic ante, she can position her shoulders on the edge of the bed and throw her head backward for a tingly head rush!

WHAT'S IN IT FOR HER

As you move together in rhythm, you'll create friction that warms up your clitoris. Because of this, you'll likely experience more satisfaction. Although this can be a tiring position, it's worth it because your man's penis is angled up toward your G-spot. Talk about double the pleasure! As if this isn't enough, you can also touch yourself while having sex in this position.

WHAT'S IN IT FOR HIM

Talk about a great view! And if your lover begins to touch herself? That will most likely put you over the edge! To take pressure off your balls, you can spread your legs.

17 · BACKSEAT DRIVER

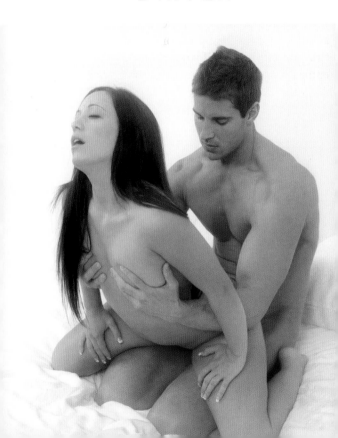

He sits with his knees in tight and tucked beneath him. She kneels in front of him so that their bodies are tucked closely together. She rubs her bottom in the area of his genitals to heat him up and then slides on top of him when they're both primed for action! This is a great position if you only have time for a quickie or if you are looking for a rear-entry position with greater potential for intimacy.

WHAT'S IN IT FOR HER
In this position, you will control the tempo of the lovemaking session, either moving quickly or slowly, thrusting your hips up and down in a circular pattern or in a gentle rocking motion. For even deeper penetration, open your legs wide. Add some oomph when you're about to come—reach behind and grasp his back to pull you both extra tight!

WHAT'S IN IT FOR HIM
Your hands will be free to roam her body, and you may want to lavish extra attention on her breasts. If you sync up with her motions, the friction and rhythm can send you both soaring!

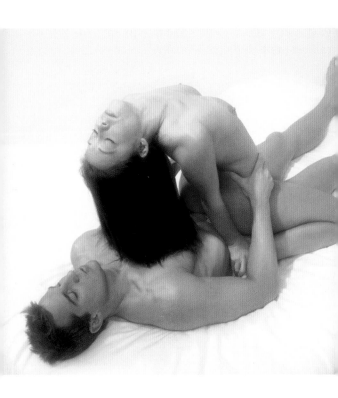

From SLICE OF HEAVEN, she can show her flexibility and maneuver into this position by leaning back and grabbing onto his ankles. He grabs her waist to control the movements, which can get pretty intense!

WHAT'S IN IT FOR HER

This is the perfect position to impart your power! You control the depth, intensity, and angle of penetration. Slow, controlled movements work best and a circular motion will get him buzzing. Deep penetration will massage your G-spot, and if you're able to free up a hand, your clitoris may also benefit from some pointed pressure!

WHAT'S IN IT FOR HIM

Since you can't see her face, you're free to let your fantasies take flight. You'll be excited to discover that "dirty" talk can ratchet up the heat! You can also caress the front of her body, play with her bottom, or reach around to finger her sweet spot.

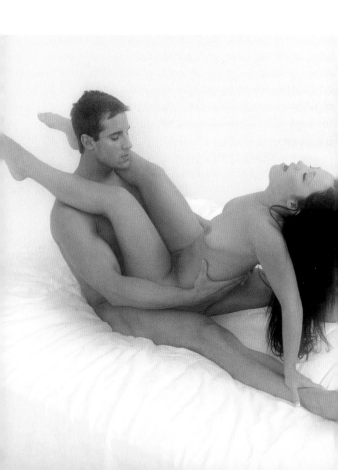

He sits up on the bed, leaning against the wall or headboard for support. She faces him and lowers herself onto his erect penis, leaning back for support, either resting her hands on the bed or grasping her man's lower legs. With his help, she raises her sexy legs up one at a time and rests them on his shoulders. In this position, movement will most likely be limited. He cradles her lower back for support and both lovers blissfully either rocking in sync together or if they're feeling especially frisky, they can take the reins and pimp his love muscle until they're both in a frenzy.

WHAT'S IN IT FOR HER

If intimacy is what you're after, this position provides plenty of opportunity. The lovemaking will be slow and sensual and may free up your lover's hand to roam to your sweet spot!

WHAT'S IN IT FOR HIM

You will relish the highly erotic nature of this pose, especially if she flaunts her body. In addition to seeing her open, you will have the perfect view of her bobbing breasts and the motion of penetration.

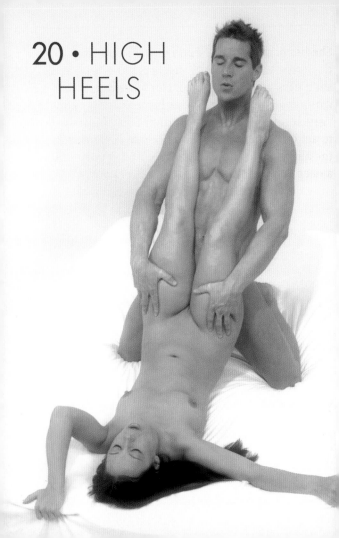

20 • HIGH HEELS

She lies back on the bed and gets into position to do a shoulder stand, with just her upper back and shoulders touching the bed. Her lover kneels in close to her and enters her as he rests her legs up against his torso. A little coordination is necessary to achieve penetration, but once you've figured out the alignment, hold on tight, because you are in for a deep ride!

WHAT'S IN IT FOR HER

You've got to be supple and flexible for this position, but there will be blissful benefits. When your legs are up, penetration is deeper during sex. That, combined with the amplified pleasure when blood rushes to your head during orgasm, will leave you feeling giddy!

WHAT'S IN IT FOR HIM

What a vista! A bit of deliberate movement is required to get into this position, so it's not likely she'll find herself in it often. You'll be especially turned on by the unique view of her elongated body. The deep penetration ensures that every inch of your penis will receive stimulation.

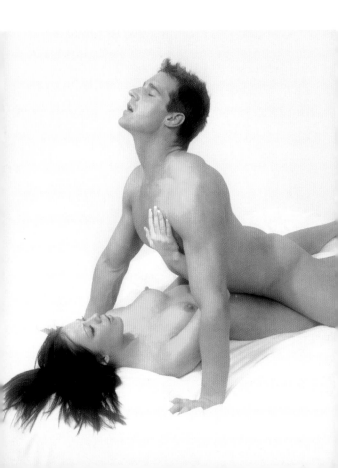

This is a twist on the missionary position. After he enters her, she pulls her legs together tightly, essentially sandwiching his penis and adding delicious friction with each thrusting motion.

WHAT'S IN IT FOR HER

The tight squeeze and genital contact of this pose mean that each time he thrusts, the pressure of his pelvis and the angle of entry will stimulate your clitoris and the sensitive nerve endings in the outer region of your vagina. This is an excellent position to move to after you've already reached orgasm, because there's a good chance your man won't be able to hold out for long!

WHAT'S IN IT FOR HIM

The tight, warm grip around your penis will have you throbbing in ecstacy in record time.

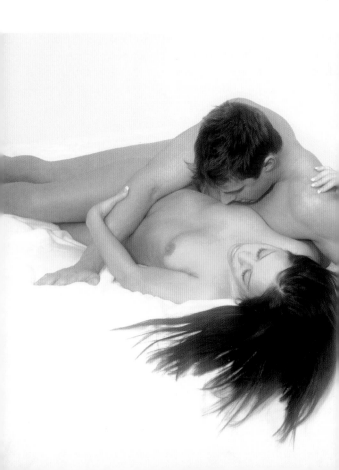

Get into the traditional spooning position: The man lies on his side with knees bent, and she also lies on her side with knees bent and her back pressed against his front. She parts her legs slightly and aligns his penis with her vagina for easy entry from the rear. She twists her upper body around to complete the spoon bender.

WHAT'S IN IT FOR HER
Full-body contact makes for highly intimate lovemaking. Penetration is shallow, so he will go for quite some time. By twisting toward your man, you will give him easier access to your breasts and clitoris.

WHAT'S IN IT FOR HIM
Before your enjoy this position, you can tease her and arouse yourself by moving your penis in and around her buttocks. Squeezing your penis between her cheeks will stimulate penetration. Once inside, you can fondle her breasts, nuzzle her neck, or whisper seductively in her ear. When she twists around, you can bite and tease her nipples.

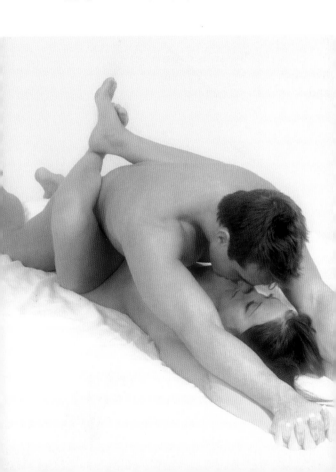

Here is a highly erotic spin on the missionary position. He mounts her as he would in the old standby, but when doing so, he pulls her arms up over her head and either holds her wrists together or lightly pins her arms down on the bed. She pulls her legs up around his back to meet his thrusting and deepen the experience.

WHAT'S IN IT FOR HER

This position is a perfect entrée into light bondage. You'll get off on him taking control of the situation. Of course, your man won't hurt you, but the feeling of being trapped may awaken latent fantasies for you. Use dirty talk to explore your desires! Keep in mind that with your legs raised around his back, you still retain some control. For added spice, pull his ass into your body by squeezing him tight!

WHAT'S IN IT FOR HIM

The thrill of domination! Under-standing that as sexual partners she trusts you enough to explore edgier ways to fulfillment.

24 · DOWNTOWN TRAIN

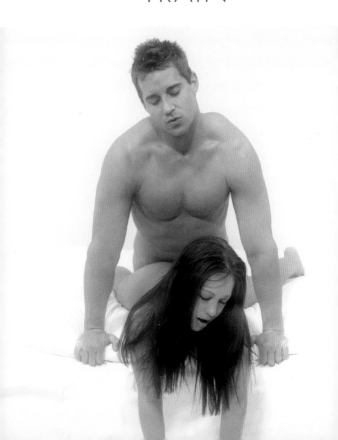

The action extends from the bed to the floor in this romp! She positions herself so that the lower half of her body (from her waist down) is on the bed and her arms are on the floor supporting her upper body, which is angled down. Her ass is right on the edge of the bed and her legs are spread open. He pulls into the station and slides in from behind. He supports his body weight by extending his arms and grasping the edge of the bed.

WHAT'S IN IT FOR HER
This position requires a bit of upper-body strength. Also, you'll need to have your man experiment with the tempo to ensure that your lovemaking session is enjoyable and not strenuous. Adding a pillow under your waist will add extra feel-good friction and all but guarantee G-spot stimulation. You'll feel extra buzzy as blood flows to your brain, making your climax even more intense!

WHAT'S IN IT FOR HIM
You'll love the feeling of control, as you pump until she can't take it any more. By just sliding to the edge of the bed, she adds a truly thrilling twist to sex.

25 • CLIT CONTROL

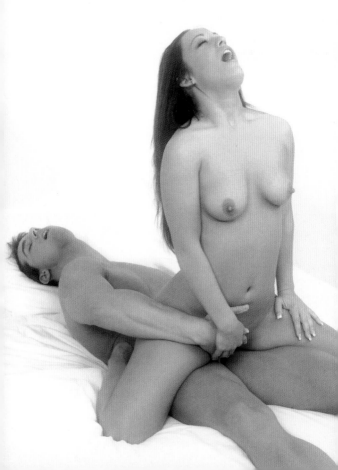

He lies on the bed and with her back to him, she slides on top of his stiff shaft. She bends her knees and places her feet behind her. She then leans back slightly so that her crown jewel is easily accessible and schools him in the fine art of pleasuring her!

WHAT'S IN IT FOR HER
You will control the tempo and intensity of thrusting. The angle of this position means his member will hit your G-spot. Moreover, you—and your man—can focus on giving you a mind-blowing orgasm by spoiling your sweet spot! If you time things just right, you can come together! At that moment, grind your hips down into his pelvis for ultra-hot sensations!

WHAT'S IN IT FOR HIM
When she leans back, your penis will go extra deep. Although this seems like a passive position for you, by pressing the right buttons you can drive her wild!

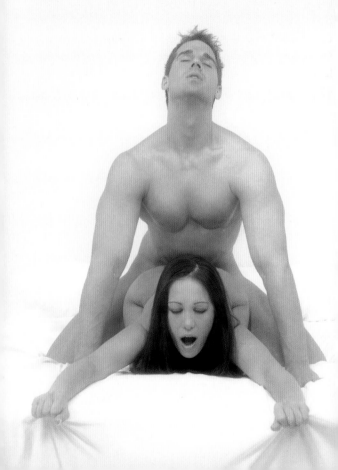

PRIMAL PUMPING is similar to RUMP ROMP, but with added animalistic eroticism. She crouches down on her knees with her arms outstretched (she can grasp the edge of the bed for the support). In a swift move, the man enters her from behind, while leaning his arms on the bed. He can pull his knees open wide for more leverage to thrust oh-so-deep!

WHAT'S IN IT FOR HER

The carnal nature of this pose brings you back to basic urges, if you're both in the mood for a rougher session. He can push well into you, so make sure the pressure is not painful. With your legs pulled into such a compact position, the added friction you feel when his privates hit your wet mound will be truly delicious!

WHAT'S IN IT FOR HIM

You are the master of your domain, and you want to take her authoritatively from behind! The sense of power combined with the exaggerated sensations that result from a tight squeeze around your throbbing member will send you over the edge!

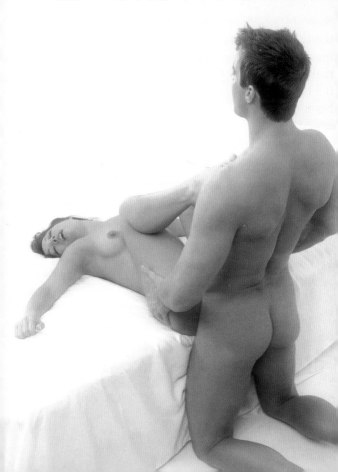

When he kneels at the alter of her sexuality, he's a changed man! She lies back with her ass near the edge of the bed. He kneels on the floor close to the edge of the bed and pulls her bent legs up to his chest. (He can put pillows under his knees to make this position more comfortable or to adjust the height.) As he gently lifts her bottom, he slides his erect penis inside of her. The result is a religious experience!

WHAT'S IN IT FOR HER
When he plays with your ass, there will be great potential for arousal. This compact pose can be made even more heavenly if you contract and release your PC muscles intermittently for an even tighter fit. While he sets the tempo, you can push against his chest and raise your bottom to meet his thrusting.

WHAT'S IN IT FOR HIM
In this position, you can feast your eyes on your erect member plunging into her willing vagina. The excitement of that combined with the pleasure that comes when she pushes against your chest will have you throbbing in no time.

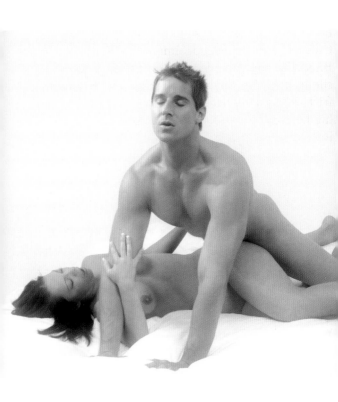

She lies on her side with her legs close together and bent at the waist (her body will almost form an L-shape). She lets her head fall back on the bed and opens her legs slightly to allow her man to enter her from behind. Similar to SPOON BENDER, but with one twist: Once he's inside, she squeezes her thighs tightly together for added friction. Crossing her legs at the ankles will help her keep them closed shut! The movement is intense—slow, gentle, and coordinated.

WHAT'S IN IT FOR HER

If you have difficulty coming without clitoral stimulation this is a great position for you! With your legs closed tight, you'll feel tingly sensations when your magic button is rubbed. The rear-entry penetration is not so much deep as it is tight. This unique angle will stimulate a new region of your vagina.

WHAT'S IN IT FOR HIM

In this position, you're better off using controlled movements, so you can savor this tight pose. You can pull yourself into a more upright position, using her bottom to support yourself. This slight variation will allow you to press her ass to deepen your thrusts.

29 • TRISEX DIPS

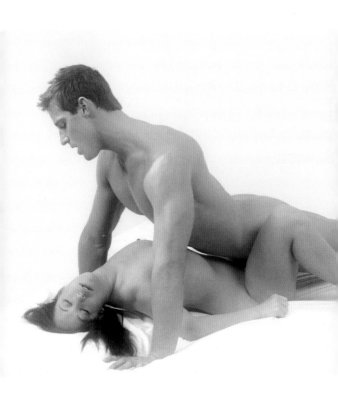

If he works hard to stay fit, this can be a sexy way for him to show off his rock-hard abs and arms while teasing her into submission! She lies on her back and he positions himself above her, as if he's going to do a push-up, balancing on the balls of his feet with his legs taut and arms fully extended near her head. As he slowly lowers himself, he uses his pelvic region to guide his erect penis into her. Balanced and controlled contact is how this position plays out, as he purposely keeps his body away from her.

WHAT'S IN IT FOR HER
This position involves genital-only contact. Agree ahead of time that you will not grab his ass, throw your legs around him, or squeeze his toned pecs. Instead, tell him in detail what you'd like to do to him, without actually doing it—if you can hold out!

WHAT'S IN IT FOR HIM
This position is deceivingly simple. When she's in such a vulnerable state it will be a challenge to resist mauling her. But it affords her the opportunity to concentrate on the sensations that build around her pelvic region when very small movements are made. You will tease her until she can't take it!

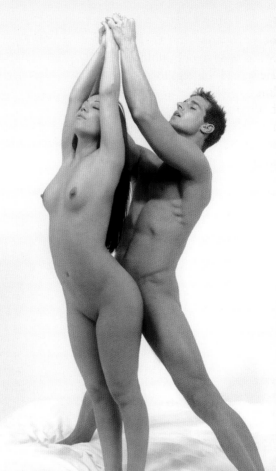

This ambitious position may be difficult for some couples to accomplish, but it's amazing what can happen when you experiment and practice it! This obviously works better if you are a similar height. Stand close to one another with the man behind. He spreads his legs to a width that puts his penis in line with the opening of her vagina. When you're both ready, he glides his erect member into her, relishing the view. He'll likely need to use his hands to do this. Once he's inside, he can raise her arms overhead and clasp hands with her. Coordinated movement is essential to finding bliss with this STANDING O.

WHAT'S IN IT FOR HER

The challenge will be remaining penetrated. You'll find that the inability to move in this pose adds an extra spark to your arousal. There are many variations: You can reach for a door jamb, lean against a wall, or use a stairway to level the playing field.

WHAT'S IN IT FOR HIM

Because of the lack of stability in this position, penetration will be shallow. Once you're inside, you may want to stay there and experiment with small circular motions and lateral jerks. The unique angle of this position may make you vulnerable to premature ejaculation, so its best used for quickies!

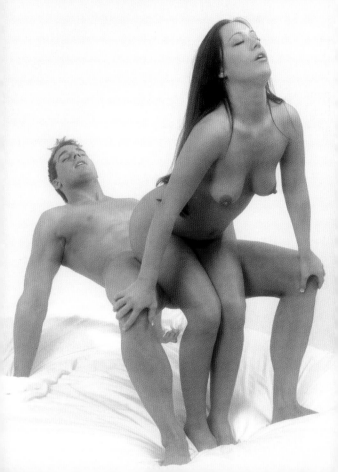

Here's a unique way to get it on—one in which the man gets a workout at the same time. He moves into a bridge-like position, with legs and arms planted firmly on the bed and his body raised so that his torso is almost entirely flat, like a table. With her back to him, she slowly sits on his erect penis, keeping her bent legs tightly together and her hands on his thighs for stability. She's in for an exciting ride in this decadent position!

WHAT'S IN IT FOR HER

The novelty of this will stay with you for quite some time! The angle allows for lots of G-spot stimulation and the friction created by your legs being closed tight will make you feel extra tingly. If you're able free up a hand, you can explore his balls and perineum. The added sensation will drive him crazy and hasten his climax.

WHAT'S IN IT FOR HIM

It may be difficult for you to maintain this position, but it won't matter because the unique angle of penetration combined with her vagina's warm and tight caress will have you ready to explode before long.

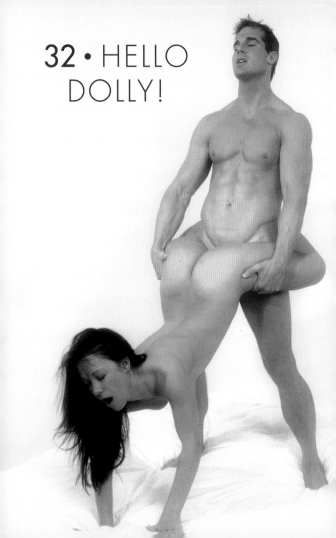

32 • HELLO DOLLY!

She positions herself on all fours either on the bed or on the floor. He stands behind and slowly grabs onto her legs, lifting them up so that they are level with his hips. At this point, she will be doing a modified handstand! He then parts her legs so he can enter her from behind. He needs to firmly grasp her upper thighs. For an added feeling of support and leverage while pumping, she can wrap the lower part of her legs around his ass.

WHAT'S IN IT FOR HER

This position requires serious arm strength, but you won't be disappointed! Penetration is deep and the angle will result in a serious G-spot massage! You'll also get the sensation of a rush of blood to the head.

WHAT'S IN IT FOR HIM

You are in absolute control of the rhythm—and anything goes! You can try circular or up-and-down motions or squeeze your legs together and then open them up. She can heighten the sensations by squeezing her PC muscles slowly and gently. Your lover can also act out as much as possible by gyrating against you while talking dirty.

33 · VALUABLE ASSETS

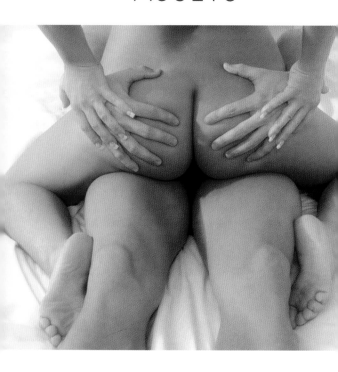

With this variation on traditional woman-on-top sex, she can begin exploring the many pleasures that can be found when she and her partner turn their attention to her ass. When they're both primed for action, she climbs on top of him and places his hands firmly on her butt cheeks. Although he probably won't need the encouragement, she can entice him to focus on her hind region with a verbal torrent of sexy commands. Be sure to be vocal about what feels good!

WHAT'S IN IT FOR HER

No matter what kind of hang-ups you might have about your ass, when your partner plays with it you'll soon forget any insecurities! In fact, inviting your man to explore your body in this way goes a long way toward becoming more comfortable in your own skin.

WHAT'S IN IT FOR HIM

Many women derive intense pleasure from having their ass grabbed, massaged, and lightly pinched, scratched, or slapped! This type of ass attention will likely fulfill some wild fantasies for both of you!

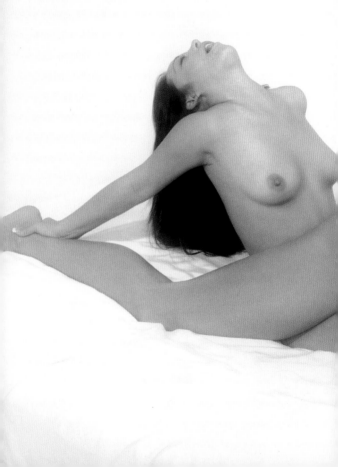

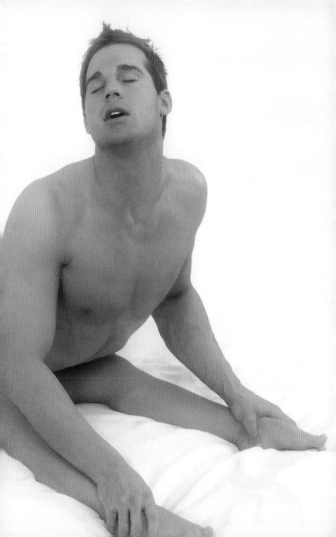

34 · RANDY ROULETTE

Here's a daring position that requires a bit of coordination. She lies on the bed with arms by her side and legs slightly parted. A pillow can be used to tilt her pelvis up for easier penetration. He is in the missionary position, but facing the opposite direction. His torso is between her legs. Once he aligns his penis, he slowly enters her and begins to work toward a rocking climax. To take this position to the next level, add a spin! When the man feels comfortable, he can begin to make his rotation around her body. She'll need to help guide his legs when they travel across her head. Unlike a roulette wheel, the spinning motion needs to be slow and controlled.

WHAT'S IN IT FOR HER

Although this position is not intimate, you can still maintain contact by either sitting up and leaning back on his legs or by lying down and grasping his buttocks. The upside will be that you get a unique view of your man's bod.

WHAT'S IN IT FOR HIM

This is a prime opportunity for you to show off your agility! Shallow thrusting will mean that the focus of penetration is on the sensitive head of your penis. An added blissful benefit is that your balls will rub against her vagina, something that feels great and doesn't always occur in tamer entanglements!

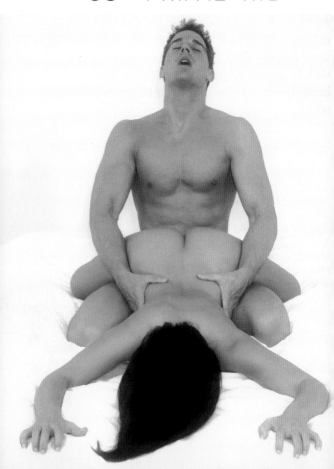

This is similar to SLICE OF HEAVEN except that the man gets to be in control! She kneels on the bed with her torso lowered and her arms extended in front of her. He also kneels, but upright. He positions himself behind his lover with his legs between hers and enters her from behind, grabbing her waist to pull her into him with each lusty thrust!

WHAT'S IN IT FOR HER
In this position, he will be perfectly angled to hit your oh-so-sensitive G-spot! Placing pillows underneath your pelvis will enhance your excitement, as each thrust creates feel-good friction on your clitoris.

WHAT'S IN IT FOR HIM
That view! Her ass and back will be on a platter for you to admire. You can grab and fondle her backside or massage and lightly scratch her back. If you're both feeling especially frisky, you can gently tug on her hair or push her arms down so that she is pinned down. In this easy-to-maneuver position, a little imagination goes a long way!

36 · SPOONFUL OF SUGAR

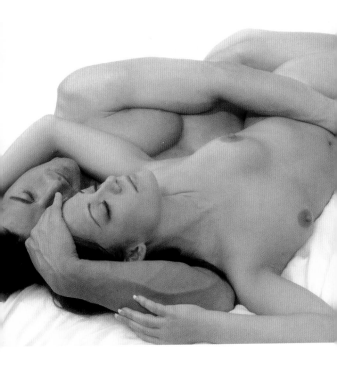

For those quieter times when you want to savor your partner in a more deliberate and loving manner, this position is a must. She lies on her side in front of her man and parts her legs slightly so he can push his erect penis into her from behind. You slowly rock to orgasm while focusing on the warm feeling of his hands exploring every inch of her body.

WHAT'S IN IT FOR HER

This highly intimate position will allow him to express his feelings for you through slow and sensuous caressing. A woman's neck is a highly erogenous area of her body, and when he's nuzzled up next to you, he's perfectly situated to tease, lick, and kiss this sensitive yet often ignored area.

WHAT'S IN IT FOR HIM

All of this touching will send a rush of feel-good chemicals to the pleasure center of your brain. By spending time exploring her body, you will become intimately acquainted with what she likes! Tell her not to be shy when it comes to telling you which buttons to push and where to linger.

37 • ROCKING HORSE

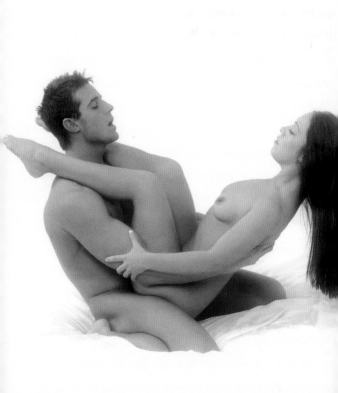

When you're in the mood for a G-spot special, the ROCKING HORSE delivers. He kneels on the bed with his legs bent underneath him. (If his knees bother him, he can extend his slightly bent legs out in front of him, instead.) Facing him, she sits down on his lap with her feet on the bed and guides his hard penis into her vagina. He grasps her back to support her. She can lean her hands back on the bed for extra support and slowly brings her legs up to rest on his shoulders. She can either remain leaning back or grab hold of his forearms. Sync your rhythm so that you're moving back and forth together.

WHAT'S IN IT FOR HER

He's not likely to come too quickly, so he will be free to focus on your pleasure! If you feel supported enough with one arm, he can free up a hand to massage your clitoris. Motion will be limited, so your man needs to gently roll his hips and sway forward and back to maintain penetration.

WHAT'S IN IT FOR HIM

You'll direct the movement, and she'll rely on your strength to keep you both balanced and in sync. You'll hold out for a long time, like a stud. If she wants to make this a more amped-up sex session, she can lean back with her hands on the bed. This will allow you to thrust even deeper.

38 · CARNAL CROSSBOW

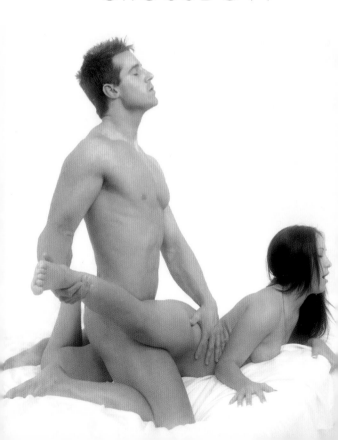

She lies on her stomach while he positions himself between her legs—they're parted like scissors. He kneels and straddles one of her legs. As he enters her from behind, he lifts her other leg so that it's fully extended. He supports her leg at the ankle while placing a hand on her hip to direct his love arrow!

WHAT'S IN IT FOR HER

If you like feeling submissive, this is a good position to try! He will drive the motion, thrust, and tempo. There's a slight angle to penetration and thrusting will be shallow, so you're in for a treat! For additional leverage, push off the side of the bed and grind into your man's pelvis.

WHAT'S IN IT FOR HIM

Your virility will be on display as you go in for the kill. You can adjust her leg height according to what feels best and pull her into you with some force. This position lends itself to role playing, so let your imagination go wild. You'll hold out for a long time, so play with it!

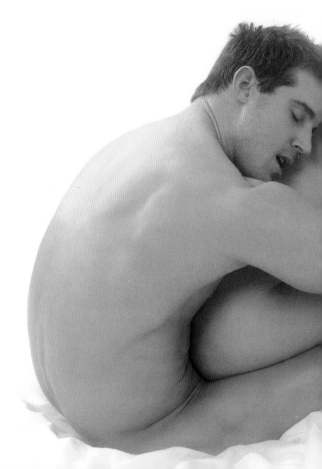

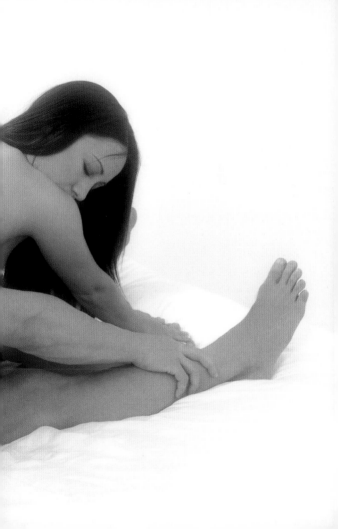

39 • FOLD & FONDLE

Although FOLD & FONDLE provides a mellow alternative to some of the more energetic positions, it's no less satisfying and makes for a great addition to your lovemaking lineup. The man sits upright on the bed with his legs outstretched in front of him. She sits on his erect penis and then slowly leans forward. He folds forward with her, as if the two of them are riding together in a toboggan. The motion is very gentle—virtually devoid of thrusting. Make waves by focusing on small, but stimulating circular gyrations and pulsing PC contractions. It may seem simple, but don't underestimate the power of the subtle application of pressure! Sync up your breathing for a truly relaxing and spiritual experience.

WHAT'S IN IT FOR HER

If you're craving intimacy, you will get it here. With your man cuddled in close, there will be some extra skin-time. He can also lavish your breasts with attention. You call the shots, so tease him by squeezing and contracting your pelvic floor—the sensation will drive him wild!

WHAT'S IN IT FOR HIM

When she leans forward, your penis will get a squeeze. Add to that the pleasure of her gripping your throbbing member and it'll be too much to handle! She can send you to the moon by fondling your testicles. The lack of movement means you're free to caress her breasts and lavish her with kisses.

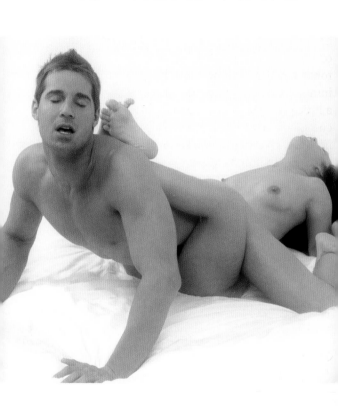

The woman lies on the bed, propping herself up on her elbows with her legs open wide. (For easier penetration, she may want to slide a pillow beneath her.) He faces away from her and positions himself on all fours, bringing his legs on either side of her torso. Once he's comfortable, he guides his penis into her vagina. Getting the angle right might take a little practice, so be sure to help each other by communicating throughout. This entanglement is pretty advanced, so make sure you relish your sexual adventurousness!

WHAT'S IN IT FOR HER

In this position, you'll receive ample stimulation in your mid-section as your clitoris and lips are in full contact with your man's pelvis and the area around his penis. The sensations concentrated around your vagina will be intense! When you use your feet and arms as leverage to pull your man in deeper, you'll be riding the big kahuna in no time!

WHAT'S IN IT FOR HIM

Embrace the rip curl for the best results (read: circular movements will get you far!). The inability to see each other makes this position exciting, as does the novelty of receiving unexpected caresses.

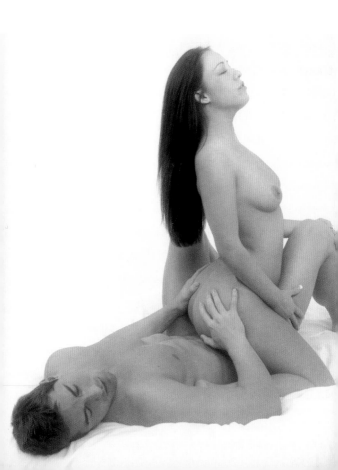

He lies on his back, with both legs slightly bent and pointing upward. She straddles his body sideways, mounting his erect penis when doing so. She uses her knees to keep herself stable. She turns her back slightly so that it is angled toward his face, and she takes him for one wild ride!

WHAT'S IN IT FOR HER

You take hold of the reins in this lusty position! You will determine the tempo, depth, and motion. Try teasing him by pulling yourself up high so that his penis is hovering at the entrance then circle around and plunge deep. Or, gyrate for a minute then switch to quick up-and-down movements, then go deep.

WHAT'S IN IT FOR HIM

You get to lie back and enjoy the ride! If you're feeling frisky, you can raise your pelvis to add a little bucking action, but otherwise you can just relish the view of her bobbing ass. She's directing this horse, and you're going wherever she points you.

42 · SIZZLING SCISSORS

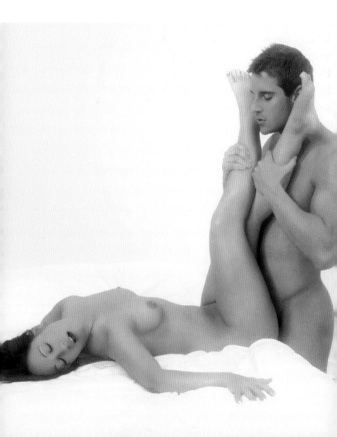

She lies on her back so that her ass is in line with the edge of the bed. She holds her legs up straight in the air. He kneels at the foot of the bed and places a pillow underneath his knees for a comfier ride, as well as adjustment of the height so that he can easily penetrate her. After entering her wet vagina, he grabs her legs, crosses them, and holds them in front of his face. He continues to crisscross her legs throughout the SIZZLING SCISSORS sex session!

WHAT'S IN IT FOR HER

The yummy sensations of your vagina squeezed tight alternated with the deep thrusting when you're spread wide open, will send a chill up your spine. Allow your hands to travel to your breasts or clitoris for additional tactile pleasures.

WHAT'S IN IT FOR HIM

If you're a leg-man this is a terrific position for you. You can tease her by telling her exactly what you'd like to do with her breasts. If you're lucky, she'll provide extra sensory stimulus by playing with herself. You'll enjoy the athletic crisscross maneuvering required to pump your penis until it's perfectly primed for climax.

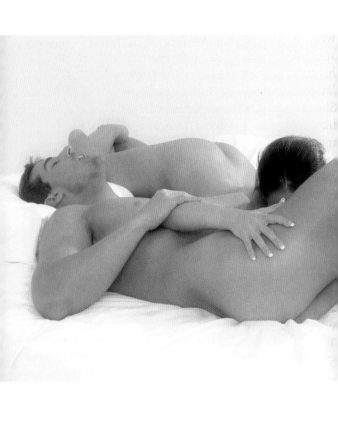

During a heated session in the sack, she pretends she is a genie and assumes her man has wished for a mind-blowing climax! She starts by spoiling him with an all-over body massage complete with special oil to relax him and release the tension in his tight muscles. He lies on his stomach, and she lavishes his back, ass, and legs with attention. She can vary the pressure and ask him what he likes best! He then flips over, and she begins by massaging his chest in a sensuous and drawn-out fashion, building up to the main event! Eventually she inches down to his pelvic region, where she focuses her erotic energies on making his dream(s) come true!

WHAT'S IN IT FOR HER
You will deliver a blissful treat!

WHAT'S IN IT FOR HIM
You receive a delicious memory that will linger in your mind—and on your body!

44 · QUEEN FOR A DAY

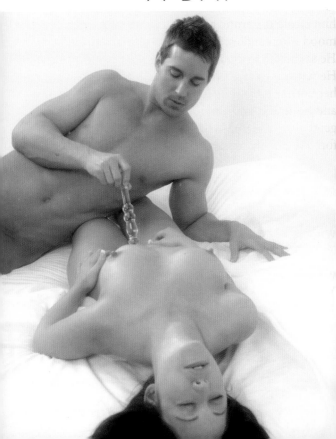

When he lavishes her with this kind of attention, she'll wonder who died and made her Queen! She sets the tone with a few royal commands (namely, "Don't dive straight for my clitoris!"), but then lets him create the erotic scene. He evokes a sensual mood with candles, pillows, aphrodisiacs, or oils. He spends time kissing her lips, breasts, and belly. He strokes her lightly with his fingertips and tells her how beautiful she is. After she's feeling relaxed and primed, he moves down between her legs and gently blows, strokes, and nibbles his way to her forbidden fruit.

WHAT'S IN IT FOR HER
Your every wish will be his command.

WHAT'S IN IT FOR HIM
You will become a valued member of the court's "inner circle."

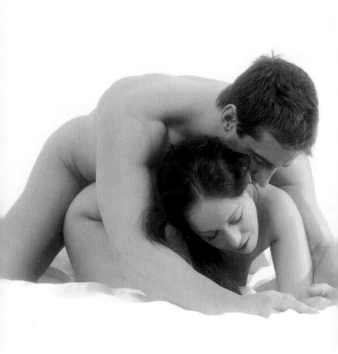

Have your fantasies ready to share, because it's confession time! While crouching on the bed, he enters her from behind and covers her with his hot bod. As his captive audience, he's free to titillate her with his innermost desires.

WHAT'S IN IT FOR HER
Hot sex with the added jolt that comes with sharing something as intimate as a fantasy.

WHAT'S IN IT FOR HIM
You can begin to broach the subject of kinkier sex in a way that will make you more willing to experiment.

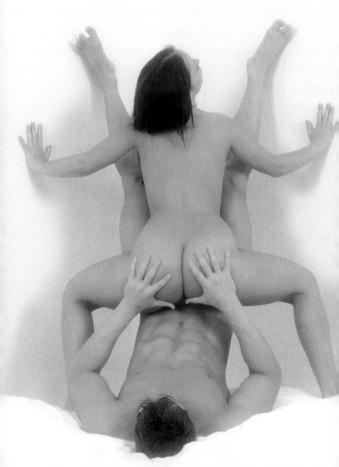

A little dexterity goes a long way toward adding spice to your sex life—this position is a testament to that. He lies down with only his head, shoulders, and upper back on the bed; his legs are upright and leaning against the wall. She positions herself so that her back is to him, and using the wall for support, squats onto his erect penis. Penetration is controlled, but then he can grab her ass and get down to the thrusting action.

WHAT'S IN IT FOR HER
Show off your hot bod, as he feels you up in any way that he pleases! In this position, his penis will rub against the front of your vaginal wall, where the elusive G-spot lives. Because you're standing, you're in the driver's seat and thrusting is easy. Grind your bottom half into your man then reach for his balls. He won't know what hit him!

WHAT'S IN IT FOR HIM
You will work a little harder than in a prone position, but the view and the tingly sensations that come from the inversion will make it all worthwhile.

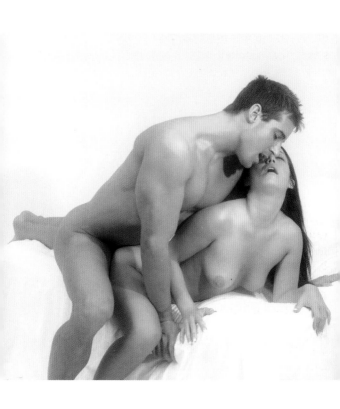

He lies face down, leaning over the edge of the bed. One leg rests on the floor and the other is outstretched. He gets into the same position, on top of her, and enters her from behind for a steamy half-on, half-off the bed romp.

WHAT'S IN IT FOR HER
Ideal for vigorous sex and deep penetration, with the added benefit of having the leverage of a foot on the floor to thrust even more energetically! His penis will hit your all-important G-spot and the animalistic nature of this sexual experience will rev both of your engines for kinkier fare.

WHAT'S IN IT FOR HIM
You'll like this position, because you will feel a sense of domination. You'll enjoy the feeling of your balls slapping against her. You can also see all of the action, which includes a sweet view of her swinging breasts.

48 · SPLITTING WOOD

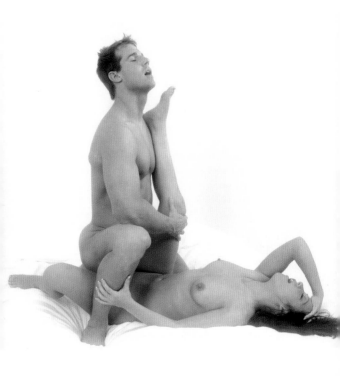

She lies on her back with one leg raised high in the air. He straddles her leg, gently enters her, and brings her raised leg to rest on his chest. (A pillow under her ass will give him a better angle to guide his penis into her vagina and achieve deeper penetration.) In this position, he can use her leg as an exciting way to leverage the many hot and heavy thrusting possibilities.

WHAT'S IN IT FOR HER

Here's a way you can show off your sexy legs! This position will allow you to flaunt your flexibility, athleticism, and sexiness. Pamper your feet beforehand, because your man will have an up-close, which is a bonus if he's got a thing for feet . . . .

WHAT'S IN IT FOR HIM

You're in control in this lusty leg-raiser! You'll be thrilled at the deep penetration, as well as turned on by the view of your erect penis disappearing into her wet vagina. You can grab her ass to pull her into you as your bodies meet during thrusting. This is one position where your animalistic side can roam free.

49 • UP & AWAY

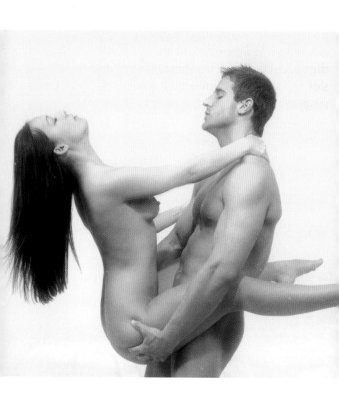

In this position, he stands. She wraps her arms around his neck, and with help from him, she wraps her legs around his waist, lining her vagina up with his penis so that he can enter her. This obviously requires strength and coordination on the part of both lovers. Maneuver into this position slowly. Once she's comfortably penetrated, let the swinging begin!

WHAT'S IN IT FOR HER
Having your man carry you in his arms can be a powerful turn-on for a woman! Sex in this position can also lend itself to very romantic, spontaneous sex. You'll feel an intimate bond with your lover as you cling to him with each swinging thrust.

WHAT'S IN IT FOR HIM
You'll relish the animalistic nature of UP & AWAY! It will also afford you the deep penetration that you've come to love. This is one position where you can show off your strength and prowess. It is both intimate and primal—the perfect combination to satisfy both partners.

50 · CROSSLEG
CANOODLE

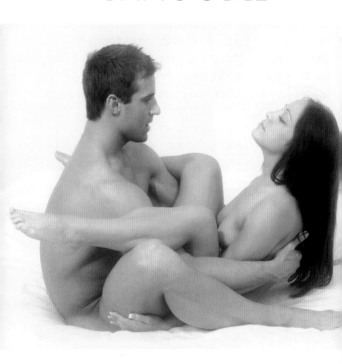

This position begins as a tangle of limbs and ends in rhythmic bliss. She starts out by straddling her man who's on his back. Her legs are bent and her feet are flat on the bed, as she slides on to his erect penis. Once they're joined, he slowly sits upright and bends his knees so that they are pointed slightly outward at a 45 degree angle. She matches his leg position and weaves her arms underneath his knees so that her hands are resting on his thighs. He does the same, but his arms come under her knees and rest on her back for support. They can hold this position for a minute and then get in sync to rock away!

WHAT'S IN IT FOR HER
Because this position is better suited for shallow penetration, your man will wake up the nerve endings in the first third of your vagina while stimulating the ultra-sensitive head of his penis—a treat for you both!

WHAT'S IN IT FOR HIM
You'll savor the wonderful close-up view of her body rubbing next to yours! Since deep thrusting may cause you to lose penetration, she can treat you to some squeezes of her PC muscles for added pleasure! Pulling her close to kiss and nuzzle her neck will elevate the experience to unforgettable.

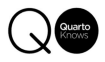

First published in the USA in 2015 by
Quiver, an imprint of
Quarto Publishing Group USA Inc.
100 Cummings Center
Suite 406-L
Beverly, MA 01915-6101
www.QuartoKnows.com
Visit our blogs at www.QuartoKnows.com

The Publisher maintains the records relating to images in this book required
by 18 USC 2257. Records are located at Quarto Publishing Group USA, Inc.
100 Cummings Center, Suite 406-L, Beverly, MA 01915-6101.

19 18 17   6 7 8 9 10

ISBN: 978-1-59233-666-1

Library of Congress Cataloging-in-Publication Data available

Cover design by traffic
Photography by Allan Penn Photography

Printed and bound in Hong Kong